RESUSCITATION:

Key data

THIRD EDITION

M. J. A. Parr
MB BS MRCP (UK) FRCA
Consultant in Anaesthesia and Intensive Therapy, Sydney, Australia

T. M. Craft
MB BS FRCA
Consultant in Anaesthesia and Intensive Care, Royal United Hospital, Bath, UK

Consultant Editor:

P. J. F. Baskett
MB BCh BAO MRCP (UK) FRCA
Past Chairman of the European Resuscitation Council, Editor of Resuscitation
Consultant Anaesthetist, Frenchay Hospital, Bristol, UK

©BIOS Scientific Publishers Limited, 1994, 1995, 1998

First published 1994 (ISBN 1 872748 53 8)
Second Edition 1995 (ISBN 1 85996 060 X)
Third Edition 1998 (ISBN 1 85996 067 7)

A CIP catalogue record for this book is available from the British Library.

ISBN 1 85996 067 7

BIOS Scientific Publishers Limited
9 Newtec Place, Magdalen Road, Oxford OX4 1RE, UK
Tel: +44 (0)1865 726286. Fax: +44 (0)1865 246823
World Wide Web home page: http://www.bios.co.uk/

DISTRIBUTORS

Australia and New Zealand
  Blackwell Science Asia
  54 University Street
  Carlton, South Victoria 3053

India
  Viva Books Private Limited
  4325/3 Ansari Road, Daryaganj
  New Delhi 110002

Singapore and South East Asia
  APAC Publishers Services
  Block 12 Lorong Bakar Batu #05–09
  Kolam Ayer Industrial Estate
  Singapore 348745

USA and Canada
  Bios Scientific Publishers
  PO Box 605, Herndon
  VA 20172–0605

Production Editor: Fran Kingston

Typeset by Richard Lloyd, Devon, UK

Printed by Biddles Ltd, Guildford, UK

Important Note from the Publisher

Contents

Contents

Contents

Abbreviations

ABG	Arterial blood gas
AED	Automatic external defibrillator
ALS	Advanced life support
BLS	Basic life support
BSA	Body surface area
CI	Cardiac index
CNS	Central nervous system
CO	Cardiac output
CPR	Cardiopulmonary resuscitation
CT	Computered tomography
CVP	Central venous pressure
CXR	Chest X-ray
ECG	Electrocardiogram
FBC	Full blood count
FiO_2	Fractional inspired oxygen concentration
GCS	Glasgow coma score
Hct	Haematocrit
ICP	Intracranial pressure
i.m.	Intramuscular
IPPV	Intermittent positive pressure ventilation
i.v.	Intravenous
MAP	Mean arterial pressure
MI	Myocardial infarction
PEF	Peak expiratory flow
PTS	Paediatric trauma score
RBC	Red blood cell
U&E	Urea and electrolytes
VF	Ventricular fibrillation
VT	Ventricular tachycardia
WBC	White blood cell

Preface to the third edition

Since the publication of the second edition of *Resuscitation: key data* there have been huge strides made towards the standardization of resuscitation techniques throughout the world. Consensus agreements have been reached through the membership of the International Liaison Committee on Resuscitation (ILCOR). This in turn has led the European Resuscitation Council to review its own guidelines for the resuscitation of both adult and paediatric patients and, in 1998, to produce recommendations which are consistent with the advisory statements of ILCOR.

At the same time we have seen the introduction of automated external defibrillators and the re-emphasis of the importance of early defibrillation in the chain of survival for victims of cardiac arrest due to ventricular fibrillation or ventricular tachycardia.

These developments and our desire to keep *Resuscitation: key data* as current as possible have led to the publication of a third edition. We have taken the opportunity to revise and update all sections of the book, whether or not they are the subject of ILCOR advisory statements or ERC guidelines. Once again we are indebted to those who have provided invaluable critique of the second edition and we hope that this book will continue to be of use to all of us working with acutely ill patients.

Michael J. A. Parr
Timothy M. Craft

Preface to the second edition

Our understanding about the processes of resuscitation and recommendations about the practical techniques involved continue to be refined. The European Resuscitation Council (ERC) have recently issued guidelines for the resuscitation of children and of adults in pre-arrest rhythms. In this, the second edition of *Resuscitation: key data*, we have included these guidelines from the ERC as well as new areas such as the resuscitation of both adults and children who are choking.

We are grateful to those of our colleagues who have provided us with invaluable feedback about the first edition and hope that this book will continue to be of help to all those involved in the resuscitation of patients young and old.

Michael J. A. Parr

January 1995   *Timothy M. Craft*

Preface to the first edition

This book contains key information for anyone involved in the resuscitation of patients. It has been collated by the authors during their practice of medicine, intensive care, and anaesthesia and includes the latest recommendations from bodies such as the European Resuscitation Council and the Resuscitation Council (UK).

Treatment of patients in an emergency situation does not afford the resuscitator the luxury of time for deliberation and discussion. It is essential, therefore, that certain data are immediately to hand.

This book includes many protocols, flow diagrams, and decision trees that have been derived from information disseminated during training courses such as those for Basic Cardiac Life Support (BCLS), Advanced Cardiac Life Support (ACLS), Advanced Trauma Life Support (ATLS), Paediatric Advanced Life Support (PALS), and Advanced Paediatric Life Support (APLS). We commend these courses and *Resuscitation: key data* is in no way designed to replace the invaluable experience that can be gained from them. The protocols should not, however, be construed as prohibiting flexibility where appropriate.

The final section of the book contains normal values for a range of investigations. Included here is ample space for the reader to make notes and record *aides-mémoires* that will result in a personalized book that is truly indispensible.

A common theme running throughout all resuscitation guidelines is the need to call for help at the earliest opportunity and this cannot be stressed enough.

Michael J. A. Parr
January 1994 *Timothy M. Craft*

Acknowledgements

We would like to acknowledge the generosity of the following who gave permission for their figures to be reproduced within this book:

The European Resuscitation Council (pp. 7, 11, 61, 65)
Resuscitation, 1998; **37** (2). In press.

The European Resuscitation Council (pp. 13–15)
Resuscitation, 1996; **31**:281.

Dr G Burton and Schwarz Pharma Ltd (pp. 18–19)

Dr P Oakley (pp. 68–69)

The British Medical Association (pp. 75)
ABC of Major Trauma. London: British Medical Association, 1991.

Surgery, Gynecology & Obstetrics (p. 79)
Surgery, Gynecology & Obstetrics, 1944; **79**:352–358.

Foreword to the third edition

The third edition of *Resuscitation: key data* includes, in addition to an update of the various key data sections, the new ERC guidelines on basic and advanced life support. These guidelines have been evolved in 1997 on the basis of policy statements published by the International Liason Committee on Resuscitation (ILCOR)

The new guidelines have been presented by the European Resuscitation Council at its biennial meeting, Resuscitation '98 held in Copenhagen in May 1998, and have, in parallel, been published in a special edition of the journal *Resuscitation*.

The new guidelines are offered as "model guidelines" to the resuscitation councils of all European countries to serve as an authoritative supranational European model. This, in turn, may be adopted in toto by the European councils or adapted as required for specific national guidelines where medicolegal, ethical, religious or medical considerations call for local variations. These variations must, however, be approved by the ERC in order to carry its logo and name.

One of the most important aims of the guidelines is to simplify the action plans to the greatest possible extent, concentrating on a single algorithm for each plan. This may facilitate European resuscitation councils to make teaching and training in basic as well as in advanced CPR simpler, more effective and, at the same time, more attractive to both lay persons and professionals

Another new chapter included in this edition is dedicated to automatic defibrillation, which may be considered as a valuable tool for first responder defibrillation programmes.

Foreword to the third edition

This book thus not only provides updated information on the sections included in the previous editions, but also introduces new guidelines on specific aspects of CPR, which have been developed with the intention of providing information based on scientific evidence instead of on unproven beliefs. This book makes the extensive experience of the authors available to a large number of health care providers involved in acute care. Concise and easy to follow advice to junior staff members is provided and the information is based on the latest scientific recommendations.

I would like to congratulate the authors on their new edition of *Resuscitation* and I am certain that anyone actively involved in the field of resuscitation will benefit from the use of this book and find it to be an indispensible aid designed to increase their personal experience and to improve their knowledge and practical skills.

Wolfgang F. Dick, FRCA
Chairman
European Resuscitation Council

Foreword to the first edition

A patient requiring resuscitation is the single most challenging situation to face the clinician. The initial resuscitation of these patients is frequently performed by the most junior members of staff with the least experience. There is no substitute for practical, hands-on experience and the authors of this book stress this aspect. There is, however, a need for the clinician to have a compact and easily accessible source of information in these situations. This book provides that information in a clear and concise form. Flow diagrams and decision trees provide a readily accessible and user-friendly approach.

The authors have had extensive experience in these situations and the problems frequently faced by junior members of staff. The advice is clear, crisp and dogmatic, and based on the most up-to-date recommendations. It will be an invaluable *aide-mémoire* for junior medical staff, medical students, and nursing and paramedic staff involved in acute care. Don't just keep it in your pocket. Read it, use it and keep using it.

Colin Robertson, FRCP FRCS FFAEM
Formerly Chairman
Resuscitation Council (UK)

Assessment of the apparently lifeless victim

Ensure safety of rescuer and victim

Gently shake casualty's shoulders. Say in a loud voice: "Are you all right?".

If casualty responds by answering or moving:

1 Leave in the position they were found in (provided they are not in further danger). Check condition, get help if needed.

2 Reassess regularly.

If casualty is unresponsive:

1 Shout for help.

2 **ABC** (Airway, Breathing, Circulation):
If possible, leave the casualty in the position they were found in.

A Open airway by loosening tight clothing around the neck and remove any obvious obstruction from the mouth. With two fingertips under the point of the chin, lift the chin. An obstructed airway may also be relieved by backward head-tilt (try to avoid in patients with suspected spinal injury) and/or jaw thrust.

B Look, listen, and feel for breathing for 10 seconds. Look for chest movements, listen at the mouth for breath sounds, feel for moving air at your cheek.

C Assess the victim for signs of a circulation. Look for movement including breathing or swallowing. Check for a carotid pulse. Take no more than 10 seconds to do this.

Assessment of the apparently lifeless victim

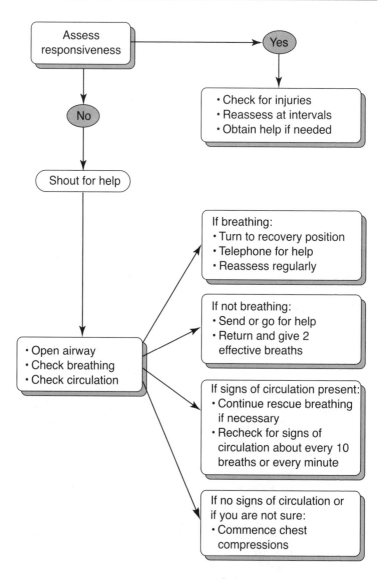

Assess responsiveness

Yes

No

- Check for injuries
- Reassess at intervals
- Obtain help if needed

Shout for help

- Open airway
- Check breathing
- Check circulation

If breathing:
- Turn to recovery position
- Telephone for help
- Reassess regularly

If not breathing:
- Send or go for help
- Return and give 2 effective breaths

If signs of circulation present:
- Continue rescue breathing if necessary
- Recheck for signs of circulation about every 10 breaths or every minute

If no signs of circulation or if you are not sure:
- Commence chest compressions

Notes: *Make no more than 5 attempts to give 2 effective breaths before checking for signs of circulation.*
In the absence of a pulse following a witnessed arrest, health care professionals may give a precordial thump before commencing chest compressions.

Basic life support (BLS)

VENTILATION

The target tidal volume for an adult is 400–600 ml.

The target rate for a victim who is not breathing but who has a pulse is 10 breaths per minute.

Inflation should take about 2 seconds.

If the victim is not breathing and has no pulse, two ventilations should be given before commencing chest compressions and then after every 15 compressions. If two rescuers are performing CPR together a single ventilation should be given after every five compressions.

CHEST COMPRESSIONS

Compressions are performed in the middle of the lower half of the sternum.

The target rate of compressions for an adult is about 100 per minute.

The sternum should be depressed by 4–5 cm during each compression.

Pressure should be applied vertically and smoothly with the same time being spent in the compressed phase as the relaxed phase.

Do not interrupt resuscitation to check for a pulse until:
➠ advanced life support has commenced
➠ the victim shows signs of life
➠ you become exhausted.

Choking – conscious

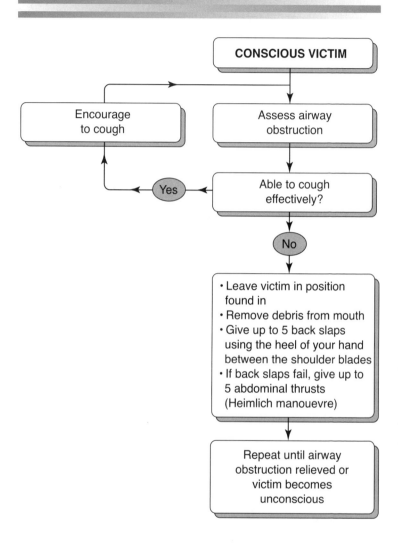

CONSCIOUS VICTIM

Encourage to cough

Assess airway obstruction

Able to cough effectively?

Yes

No

- Leave victim in position found in
- Remove debris from mouth
- Give up to 5 back slaps using the heel of your hand between the shoulder blades
- If back slaps fail, give up to 5 abdominal thrusts (Heimlich manouevre)

Repeat until airway obstruction relieved or victim becomes unconscious

Note: *The Heimlich manouevre is performed standing behind the victim with the victim bending well forward. Grasp one fist with your other hand, in the midline, slightly above the navel. Using quick inward and upward thrusts, pull your fist into the upper abdomen.*

Choking – unconscious

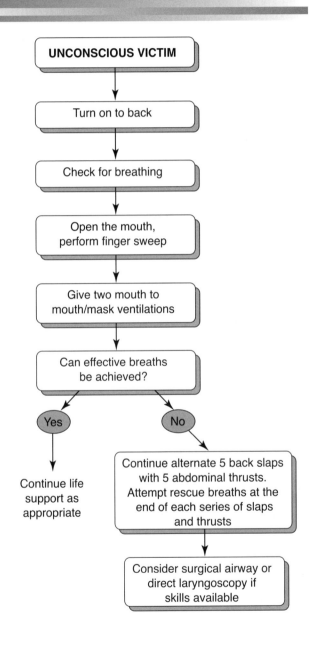

UNCONSCIOUS VICTIM

Turn on to back

Check for breathing

Open the mouth,
perform finger sweep

Give two mouth to
mouth/mask ventilations

Can effective breaths
be achieved?

Yes

No

Continue life
support as
appropriate

Continue alternate 5 back slaps
with 5 abdominal thrusts.
Attempt rescue breaths at the
end of each series of slaps
and thrusts

Consider surgical airway or
direct laryngoscopy if
skills available

Advanced life support (ALS)

The following pages contain treatment recommendations presented as algorithms.

By their very nature, algorithms over-simplify. They are not intended to replace clinical understanding or prohibit flexibility; adopting a cookbook approach to the management of acutely ill patients does not relieve the chef of the need to think.

When applying these treatment recommendations it is essential to remember that early defibrillation, adequate oxygenation and ventilation through a clear airway, and chest compressions, are always more important than the administration of drugs.

The algorithms assume that the underlying rhythm being treated persists. The treatment sequence should, of course, be interrupted at any point should the arrhythmia terminate.

Above all, **treat the patient, not the monitor.**

Note: *Defibrillators should always be charged with the paddles held against the patient's chest wall or whilst housed in the defibrillator. They should never be charged with the paddles held in the air.*

Adult cardiac arrest

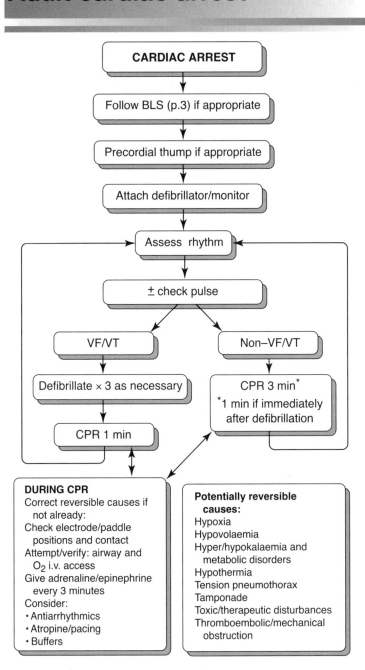

CARDIAC ARREST

Follow BLS (p.3) if appropriate

Precordial thump if appropriate

Attach defibrillator/monitor

Assess rhythm

± check pulse

VF/VT

Non–VF/VT

Defibrillate × 3 as necessary

CPR 3 min*
*1 min if immediately
after defibrillation

CPR 1 min

DURING CPR
Correct reversible causes if
  not already:
Check electrode/paddle
  positions and contact
Attempt/verify: airway and
  O_2 i.v. access
Give adrenaline/epinephrine
  every 3 minutes
Consider:
• Antiarrhythmics
• Atropine/pacing
• Buffers

**Potentially reversible
  causes:**
Hypoxia
Hypovolaemia
Hyper/hypokalaemia and
  metabolic disorders
Hypothermia
Tension pneumothorax
Tamponade
Toxic/therapeutic disturbances
Thromboembolic/mechanical
  obstruction

Ventricular fibrillation/pulse-less ventricular tachycardia

In adults, the commonest primary arrhythmia at the onset of cardiac arrest is ventricular fibrillation (VF) or pulseless ventricular tachycardia (VT). Most survivors of cardiac arrest commence with one of these rhythms.

The definitive treatment of these arrhythmias – defibrillation – must be administered promptly.

The chances of successful defibrillation decline substantially with each passing minute.

Defibrillation

The initial three shocks in the treatment sequence of any new episode of VF/VT should be delivered at 200 J, 200 J, and 360 J.

Thereafter each shock should be of 360 J.

Adrenaline/epinephrine

Adrenaline/epinephrine 1 mg i.v. should be given at the completion of each loop (rhythm assessment, defibrillation × 3, CPR for 1 min). In practice this means giving adrenaline/epinephrine every 2–3 minutes.

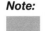

Note: *Continue loops for as long as defibrillation is indicated. After two loops consider an antiarrhythmic or alkalizing (buffer) agent.*

Non-ventricular fibrillation/ ventricular tachycardia

If VF/VT can be positively excluded, defibrillation is not indicated.

Cardiac arrest with non-VF/VT rhythms carries a less favourable prognosis. There are, however, some potentially reversible causes of non-VF/VT cardiac arrest. During the search for and treatment of these causes CPR and adrenaline/epinephrine administration should continue.

Atropine

Atropine 3 mg i.v. may be given once to a patient with non-VT/VF arrest. This dose will block vagal activity in an adult.

Note: Consider pressor agents, calcium, alkalizing agents, or 5 mg adrenaline/epinephrine.

Automatic external defibrillators

Survival from VF falls by ~7–10% for every minute after collapse. Early defibrillation is the single most important therapy for patients in VF. Automatic external defibrillators (AEDs) have been developed to permit the widest possible access to defibrillation whether by medically trained personnel or not.

An AED will accommodate the practice of either a lay first responder or fully trained ALS provider.

If an AED is immediately available, its attachment and rhythm analysis are of the utmost priority. Time should not be wasted attempting rescue breaths.

When a shock is indicated, the priority is rapid defibrillation. Checking the pulse between the first three shocks is counter-productive and should not be allowed to interfere with rhythm analysis.

After the first three shocks, uninterrupted CPR should be given for one minute (see Adult cardiac arrest algorithm, p. 7). The CPR interval will be timed by the AED.

If "No shock" is indicated (see Adult cardiac arrest algorithm, p. 7), uninterrupted CPR should be performed for three minutes. After three minutes a voice prompt from the AED will indicate that CPR should be stopped and the ANALYSE button pressed.

Further treatment will be as per the cardiac arrest algorithm and prompted by the AED.

AED Algorithm

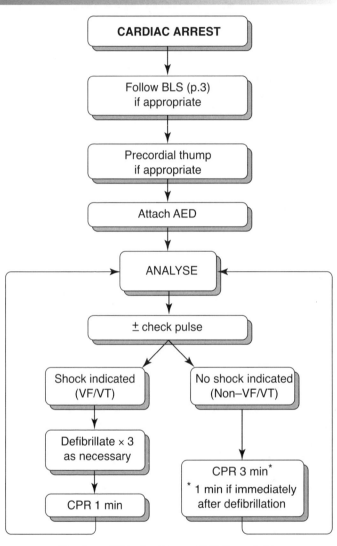

Continue AED algorithm until ALS available

Peri-arrest arrhythmias

Malignant cardiac rhythm disorders may lead to cardiac arrest or follow initial resuscitation from a cardiac arrest.

The following three algorithms are universally applicable; drugs which are not widely available in all countries have been omitted.

Stated drug doses are based on an adult of average weight.

In all circumstances it is assumed that oxygen is being given and that intravenous access has been established.

Bradycardia

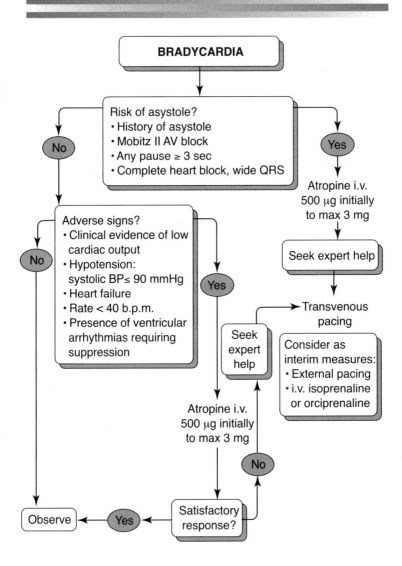

BRADYCARDIA

Risk of asystole?
- History of asystole
- Mobitz II AV block
- Any pause ≥ 3 sec
- Complete heart block, wide QRS

No

Yes

Atropine i.v.
500 μg initially
to max 3 mg

Seek expert help

Adverse signs?
- Clinical evidence of low cardiac output
- Hypotension: systolic BP ≤ 90 mmHg
- Heart failure
- Rate < 40 b.p.m.
- Presence of ventricular arrhythmias requiring suppression

No

Yes

Transvenous pacing

Seek expert help

Consider as interim measures:
- External pacing
- i.v. isoprenaline or orciprenaline

Atropine i.v.
500 μg initially
to max 3 mg

No

Observe

Yes

Satisfactory response?

Narrow complex tachycardia
(supraventricular tachycardia)

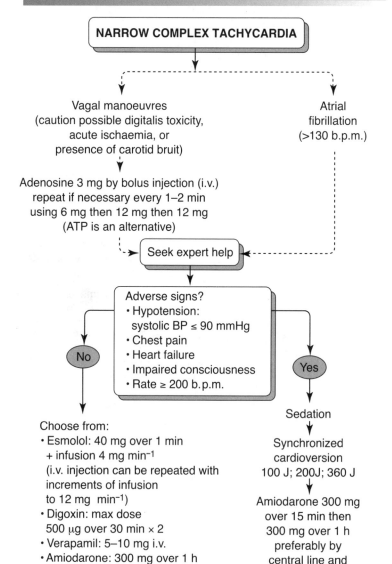

NARROW COMPLEX TACHYCARDIA

Vagal manoeuvres
(caution possible digitalis toxicity,
acute ischaemia, or
presence of carotid bruit)

Atrial
fibrillation
(>130 b.p.m.)

Adenosine 3 mg by bolus injection (i.v.)
repeat if necessary every 1–2 min
using 6 mg then 12 mg then 12 mg
(ATP is an alternative)

Seek expert help

Adverse signs?
• Hypotension:
  systolic BP ≤ 90 mmHg
• Chest pain
• Heart failure
• Impaired consciousness
• Rate ≥ 200 b.p.m.

No

Yes

Choose from:
• Esmolol: 40 mg over 1 min
+ infusion 4 mg min⁻¹
(i.v. injection can be repeated with
increments of infusion
to 12 mg min⁻¹)
• Digoxin: max dose
500 μg over 30 min × 2
• Verapamil: 5–10 mg i.v.
• Amiodarone: 300 mg over 1 h
• overdrive pacing (not AF)

Sedation

Synchronized
cardioversion
100 J; 200J; 360 J

Amiodarone 300 mg
over 15 min then
300 mg over 1 h
preferably by
central line and
repeat cardioversion

Notes: *Vagal manoeuvres include the Valsalva manoeuvre, and carotid sinus massage (performed unilaterally and only after a carotid bruit has been excluded).*
ß-blockade after verapamil may result in AV node standstill.

Broad complex tachycardia
(sustained ventricular tachycardia)

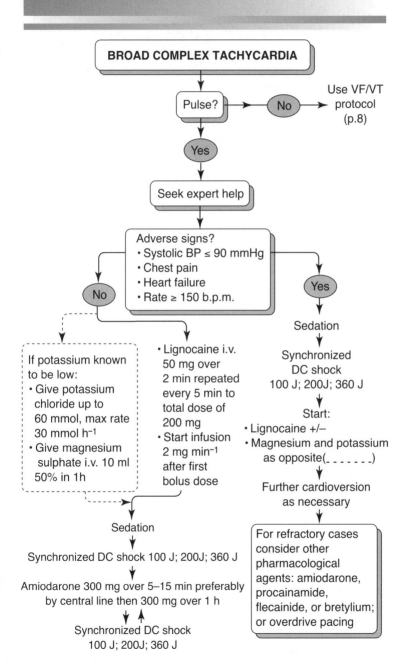

BROAD COMPLEX TACHYCARDIA

Pulse? → No → Use VF/VT protocol (p.8)

Yes

Seek expert help

Adverse signs?
• Systolic BP ≤ 90 mmHg
• Chest pain
• Heart failure
• Rate ≥ 150 b.p.m.

No

Yes

Yes branch:
Sedation

Synchronized DC shock
100 J; 200J; 360 J

Start:
• Lignocaine +/–
• Magnesium and potassium as opposite(_ _ _ _ _ _)

Further cardioversion as necessary

For refractory cases consider other pharmacological agents: amiodarone, procainamide, flecainide, or bretylium; or overdrive pacing

No branch:
If potassium known to be low:
• Give potassium chloride up to 60 mmol, max rate 30 mmol h^{-1}
• Give magnesium sulphate i.v. 10 ml 50% in 1h

• Lignocaine i.v. 50 mg over 2 min repeated every 5 min to total dose of 200 mg
• Start infusion 2 mg min^{-1} after first bolus dose

Sedation

Synchronized DC shock 100 J; 200J; 360 J

Amiodarone 300 mg over 5–15 min preferably by central line then 300 mg over 1 h

Synchronized DC shock
100 J; 200J; 360 J

Antiarrhythmic drug doses

Adenosine:

by rapid i.v. injection ....3 mg
2nd dose (if required) ....6 mg
3rd dose (if required) ....12 mg
Further dosage not recommended.

Amiodarone:

over 20–120 min (via central vein) ....5 mg kg^{-1}
max dose in 24 h..1.2g

Bretylium:

initial dose over 8–10 min ....5–10 mg kg^{-1}
repeated after 1-2 h to a total dosage of ......30 mg kg^{-1}

Digoxin:

initial i.v. dose over >1 h ....0.75–1 mg

Esmolol:

initial i.v. dose over 1 min ....500 µg kg^{-1}
followed by infusion for 4 min of..................50 µg kg^{-1} min^{-1}
The loading dose may then be repeated and the maintnance
infusion rate doubled if the response is inadequate.

Lignocaine:

initial slow bolus ....100 mg
followed by infusion of ....2–4 mg min^{-1}

Magnesium:

by slow bolus...2 g
followed by infusion of ....1 g h^{-1}
for 5–10h

Verapamil:

by slow bolus...5–10 mg

Infusion drug doses

Adrenaline/Epinephrine ....0.01–0.5 µg kg^{-1} min^{-1}

Aminophylline:
    loading dose (over 20 min) ....5 mg kg^{-1}
    followed by ....500 µg kg^{-1} h^{-1}

Dobutamine.....................................2–20 µg kg^{-1} min^{-1}

Dopamine...2–15 µg kg^{-1} min^{-1}

Dopexamine.....................................0.25–2 µg kg^{-1} min^{-1}

Glyceryl trinitrate...........................10–200 µg min^{-1}

Isoprenaline.....................................0.5–10 µg min^{-1}

Nitroprusside:
    initial rate ....0.3–1 µg kg^{-1} min^{-1}
    usual dose range ....0.5–6 µg kg^{-1} min^{-1}
    maximum dose ....8 µg kg^{-1} min^{-1}

Noradrenaline/Norepinephrine...0.01–0.5 µg kg^{-1} min^{-1}

Note: *These doses are the usual ranges and do not preclude the use of an initial bolus or much higher infusion doses in exceptional circumstances.*

Drug infusion nomograms

For solutions containing 1 mg ml^{-1} a straight line is drawn from "patient dose rate" to "body weight" and the "infusion pump rate" read from the nomogram scale.

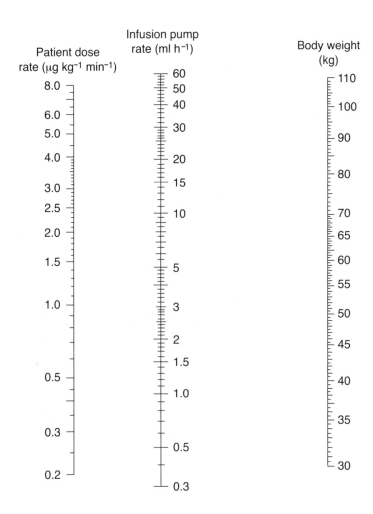

Drug infusion nomograms

Dopamine, dobutamine, or aminophylline

use 200 mg and make up with 5% glucose to a total volume as per the adjacent scale

> 1 ml h^{-1} gives
> 1.0 μg kg^{-1} min^{-1}

Sodium nitroprusside

use 50 mg and make up with 5% glucose to a total volume as per the adjacent scale

> 1 ml h^{-1} gives
> 0.25 μg kg^{-1} min^{-1}

Adrenaline/Epinephrine, noradrenaline or isoprenaline

use 5 mg and make up with 5% glucose to a total volume as per the adjacent scale

> 1 ml h^{-1} gives
> 0.025 μg kg^{-1} min^{-1}

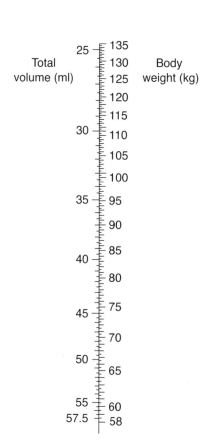

Total volume (ml)

Body weight (kg)

19

Hyperkalaemia

The ECG changes associated with hyperkalaemia include:

peaked T waves
loss of the P wave
wide, slurred QRS complex
ventricular tachycardia or fibrillation.

Emergency treatment of hyperkalaemia comprises:

1 Stop administration of potassium.

2 10 ml 10% calcium chloride i.v. (extreme caution in digitalized patients).

3 50 ml 50% glucose with 20 units of short-acting insulin followed, if necessary, by 1 litre 20% glucose with 100 units of insulin infused at 2 ml kg^{-1} h^{-1}.

4 Promote alkalinization by hyperventilation if intubated, or give i.v. sodium bicarbonate.

Chest pain and possible acute myocardial infarction

IMMEDIATE ACTIONS

➠ Oxygen
➠ Intravenous access
➠ Pain control. Diamorphine 2.5–5 mg i.v. repeated as required and an antiemetic, e.g. metoclopramide 10 mg i.v. or cyclizine 25–50 mg i.v.
➠ Aspirin 75 mg orally or 300 mg chewed then swallowed
➠ ECG (CXR later)
➠ Blood tests   FBC, U&Es, glucose, cardiac enzymes, cholesterol

URGENT THROMBOLYSIS

➠ If chest pain suggestive of myocardial infarction
   or
➠ ST elevation >0.2 mV in more than two adjacent chest leads or >0.1 mV in limb leads

Administer thrombolytic ASAP

NB do not wait for confirmatory lab results

CONSIDER

➠ β-blockade
➠ Heparin s.c.

Chest pain and possible acute myocardial infarction

THROMBOLYSIS

Indications

Patients within 24 h of major symptoms suggestive of acute myocardial infarction. ECG changes of ST elevation >0.2 mV in more than 2 adjacent chest leads or >0.1 mV in limb leads.

Absolute contraindications

Active haemorrhage. Recent CNS infarction, haemorrhage, surgery, trauma, or malignancy.

Relative contraindications

Recent non-CNS surgery (<10 days). Recent trauma (<10 days). Recent gastrointestinal haemorrhage. Recent external cardiac massage. Coagulation disorders. Pregnancy or <10 days post partum. Severe hypertension (diastolic >130 mmHg).

Drugs

1 **Streptokinase** – for almost all patients

1.5 mega units in 0.9% sodium chloride given over 60 mins.

2 **tPA** with intravenous heparin if:

➡ streptokinase given within 5 days–12 months previously
➡ patient aged <75 years, large anterior MI, within 4 h of onset of symptoms
➡ severe persistent hypotension especially if aggravated by streptokinase

give 15 mg i.v. bolus, then infusion of 0.75 mg kg^{-1} over 30 mins (max 50 mg), then 0.5 mg kg^{-1} over 60 mins (max 35 mg).

Normal ECG values

The standard speed for recording an ECG is 25 mm sec^{-1}.

At this rate one large square represents 0.2 sec.

At this rate one small square represents 0.04 sec.

Every ECG should be calibrated vertically; two large squares = 1 mV.

NORMAL ADULT VALUES

Rate .... $60–100 \text{ min}^{-1}$
PR interval .... 0.12–0.20 sec
P wave – maximum height: .... 2.5 mm
              – maximum duration: .... 0.11 sec
QRS   – axis: .... -30° to +90°
              – duration: .... <0.1 sec
QT_C (corrected for heart rate): .... <0.42 sec

Normal cardiac and haemodynamic values

MAP	70–105 mmHg
CVP	0–7 mmHg
MPAP	9–16 mmHg
PAOP	8–12 mmHg
CO	$4-8 \text{ l min}^{-1}$
CI	$2.5-4 \text{ l min}^{-1} \text{m}^{-2}$
SV	$60-130 \text{ ml beat}^{-1}$
LVSWI	$44-68 \text{ g-m m}^{-2} \text{beat}^{-1}$
RVSWI	$4-8 \text{ g-m m}^{-2} \text{beat}^{-1}$
PVR	$25-125 \text{ dyn sec}^{-1} \text{cm}^{-5}$
SVR	$960-1400 \text{ dyn sec}^{-1} \text{cm}^{-5}$
$(A\text{-}a)DO_2$	<3 kPa

Notes:

$(A\text{-}a)DO_2$	=	Alveolar arterial oxygen difference
CO	=	cardiac output
LVSWI	=	left ventricular stroke work index
MPAP	=	mean pulmonary artery pressure
PAOP	=	pulmonary artery occlusion pressure
PVR	=	pulmonary vascular resistance
RAP	=	right atrial pressure
RVSWI	=	right ventricular stroke work index
SVR	=	systemic vascular resistance
1 kPa	=	7.5 mmHg

Sequence of trauma management

1 Perform rapid visual scan and obtain history; simultaneously perform the primary survey.

2 **PRIMARY SURVEY AND START OF RESUSCITATION**

A **Airway** (with cervical spine control)
Relieve airway obstruction, e.g. chin lift, jaw thrust, insertion of airway, intubation, surgical airway.
Give oxygen.
Avoid nasal airways and/or nasogastric tubes if suspicion of base of skull fracture.

B **Breathing** (with ventilatory support)
Correct inadequate ventilation.
Drain pneumothorax/haemothorax.
Seal open chest wound.

C **Circulation**
Control external haemorrhage.
Site two larger than 16G i.v. cannulae and obtain blood samples.
Correct hypovolaemia with warm fluids.
Initial fluid infusion of 2–3 litres of crystalloid in adults, followed by blood if the patient is still hypotensive.

D **Disability**
Glasgow coma score (q.v.).
Assess pupil responses.
Assess limb movements.

E **Expose** completely for examination but avoid inducing hypothermia.

Sequence of trauma management

2 **PRIMARY SURVEY Cont.**

Monitoring:

ECG
Blood pressure
Temperature
Oxygen saturation by pulse oximetry
Urine output
End expired tidal carbon dioxide (if intubated)

3 **RESUSCITATION PHASE**

Continuing management of problems as they are detected in the primary survey.

4 **SECONDARY SURVEY**

Sequence of detailed head to toe examination:
Scalp and head
Maxillofacial
Eyes, ears, nose and throat
Neck and cervical spine
Chest
Abdomen
Pelvis and rectum
Extremities (vascular and musculoskeletal)
Neurological function

5 **DEFINITIVE CARE**

Procedures:

Cervical and thoracolumbar immobilization
Airway insertion; oral or nasal
Intubation; oral or nasal
Cricothyroidotomy; needle or surgical

Sequence of trauma management

Thoracocentesis; needle or chest tube
Vascular access; peripheral, central, or surgical
Pericardiocentesis
Oro/nasogastric tube
Urinary catheter
Diagnostic peritoneal lavage
Immobilization of fractures

Investigations:

Blood samples for:
FBC, U&E, X-match, ABG, alcohol, and illicit
drugs
X-rays:
lateral cervical spine from C_1 to C_7 (including the
top of T_1)
chest
pelvis
others as indicated

Notes: *Head and cervical spine immobilization is achieved by manual in-line stabilization (MILS) or semi-rigid collar with sand bags and tape.*
Thoracolumbar immobilization is achieved with the use of a long spine board.
Any evidence of a urethral injury is an indication for retrograde urethrography and is a contraindication to perurethral bladder catheterization.

Diagnostic peritoneal lavage

Lavage is performed with 10 ml kg^{-1} of lactated Ringer's solution or 0.9% saline.

The insertion site for lavage is in the midline, one-third of the distance from the umbilicus to the symphysis pubis.

POSITIVE RESULT

Aspiration of gross blood >10 ml.
Lavage fluid exits via chest tube or urinary catheter.
Lavage fluid contains:
  Evidence of food, foreign particles, faeces or bile.
  RBC >100 000 x 10^6 l^{-1} from blunt trauma.
  RBC >50 000 x 10^6 l^{-1} from penetrating trauma.
  WBC >500 x 10^6 l^{-1}.

NEGATIVE RESULT

Lavage fluid contains:
  RBC <20 000 x 10^6 l^{-1}.
  WBC <100 x 10^6 l^{-1}.

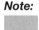

Note: *Abdominal ultrasound and CT scanning are used in some centres. Peritoneal lavage may still be helpful in the management of patients suffering multi-trauma*

Revised trauma score

		Parameter		
		GCS	BP (mmHg)	Resp. rate (min⁻¹)
Coded value	4	13–15	>89	10–29
	3	9–12	76–89	>29
	2	6–8	50–75	6–9
	1	4–5	1–49	1–5
	0	3	0	0
Score coefficient		0.9368	0.7326	0.2908
Product		A	B	C

Product = Coded value × Score coefficient

Revised trauma score = Sum of A + B + C

The sum of the resulting values ranges from 0 to 7.8408. The higher the value the better the prognosis.

Note: The score coefficient for GCS is the greatest to allow for the identification of those with a severe head injury and little physiological change.

Trauma in pregnancy

The priorities of assessment and management described earlier (pp. 25–29) also apply to pregnant victims of trauma.

Key points to remember for trauma in pregnancy:

There are two patients to consider.

Placental blood flow is compromised to maintain maternal circulation. Careful monitoring of both mother and fetus are essential for favourable fetal outcome.

Aortocaval compression is avoided by the use of left uterine displacement provided by a wedge under the right hip/spine board.

The normal hyperventilation of late pregnancy which results in a $PaCO_2$ of 4 kPa should be maintained if assisted ventilation is employed.

Diagnostic peritoneal lavage is performed in the midline above the uterus.

Emergency caesarian section may save both mother and baby.

Glasgow coma score

Behaviour	Response		score
Eye opening	Spontaneous	E	4
	To speech		3
	To pain		2
	Nil		1
Motor response	Obeys	M	6
(to verbal/painful stimulus)	Localizes		5
	Normal flexion		4
	Abnormal flexion		3
	Abnormal extension		2
	Nil		1
Verbal response	Orientated	V	5
	Confused		4
	Inappropriate		3
	Incomprehensible		2
	Nil		1

The highest score possible is 15.
The lowest score possible is 3.

Management of severe head injury

Successful outcomes from severe head injury depend upon rapid assessment and resuscitation followed by consultation with neurosurgical receiving centres and transfer of appropriate patients.

Guidelines are presented but local protocols should always be followed.

Management of seizures

⟶ Diazemuls 0.1–0.2 mg kg^{-1} plus
⟶ Phenytoin 15 mg kg^{-1} over 15 mins
⟶ Thiopentone 3 mg kg^{-1} by anaesthetist if required
⟶ recheck ABC

Management of increased ICP in intracranial haematoma pending or during transfer

⟶ Mannitol 0.5 g kg^{-1} (wt(kg) × 2.5 = ml of 20% mannitol)
⟶ manual hyperventilation (30 sec)
⟶ nurse head up 30° if possible
⟶ ensure no obstruction to venous blood flow from cervical collar

Paediatric considerations

⟶ maintain systolic BP >90 mmHg
⟶ consider intraosseous access
⟶ blood loss from scalp may be significant
⟶ child <15 kg give 4% glucose/0.18% saline
⟶ check blood sugar
⟶ beware hypothermia

Assessment and resuscitation

Airway with cervical spine control

Breathing ventilatory support

Intubation urgently if:
- airway compromise
- ventilatory failure
- GCS ≤8
- warranted because of other injury
- required to facilitate CT

Management of intubation
- rapid sequence induction with cricoid pressure and manual in-line stabilization
- maintenance anaesthesia
- neuromuscular paralysis
- ventilation to normocapnia
- orogastric tube

Anaesthetic drugs

Intubation:
- thiopentone 3–5 mg kg^{-1} or propofol 1–3 mg kg^{-1}
- suxamethonium 1–2 mg kg^{-1}
- fentanyl 2–5 μg kg^{-1}

Maintenance:
- vecuronium 0.1 mg kg^{-1} pm
- propofol infusion (1–5 mg kg^{-1} h^{-1})

Hypotension:
- consider vasopressors if hypovolaemia excluded

Circulation
control of haemorrhage
maintenance of BP

- secure i.v. access
- maintenance fluid: 0.9% saline
- systolic BP >120mmHg
  - colloid first
  - blood if required
  - vasopressor (see anaesthetic drugs)
- Hb >10g dl^{-1}
- urethral catheter

Disability
rapid assessment of GCS and pupillary responses

Exposure
complete examination and log-roll

Assess and treat extracranial injuries
- complete secondary survey as ATLS and treat as required
- cervical spine, chest and pelvic X-rays
- persistent hypotension indicates extracranial injury

Do not transfer until life-threatening extracranial injuries stable and no persistent hypotension

Decision to consult/transfer

Avoid secondary brain injury

Cause: Aim:
- hypotension   systolic BP> 120mmHg
- hypoxia $PaO_2 > 13$ kPa/$SpO_2 > 95\%$
- hyper/hypocapnia $PaCO_2$ 4.0–4.5 kPa
- raised ICP
- seizures
- hyperthermia   core temp. 35–37°c
- hyperglycaemia   BS 4–7 mmol l^{-1}

Critical:
- not obeying commands plus
- deteriorating GCS and/or
- progressive focal signs
  (motor/pupillary)

→

- immediate neurosurgical consultation
- transfer/scan as agreed
  Do not delay consultation for CT scan

Severe:
- not obeying commands but
- GCS stable
- systemically stable

→

- urgent CT scan

↓

- neurosurgical consultation with CT image-link
- transfer as appropriate

Moderate:
- obeying commands but impaired consciousness
- GCS stable

↓

- early CT scan (< 4 hours)

→

- CT scan abnormal
- clinical progress unsatisfactory
- other complications e.g. compound depressed fracture

↑

↓

- CT normal
- GCS stable/ improving
- no other complications

→

- observe and manage locally

Transfer

Inter hospital transfer
Only when cardio/resp stable
• intubated/sedated/paralysed
• check tracheal tube and i.v. access (×2)
• doctor and nurse/paramedic with appropriate experience
• monitor and record
    – SpO$_2$, BP, ECG
    – PE'CO$_2$ if possible
    – pupillary responses 1/4 hourly
• cervical spine protcetion
• treat raised ICP
• inform ICU of ETA

Check list
• adequate oxygen
• airway equipment
    – self-inflating bag
    – laryngoscope
    – tracheal tube
    – airway
    – mask
    – suction
• CT scans
• venous cannulae
• fluid
• drugs/equipment for resuscitation/anaesthesia
• mannitol

Essential information
• name, age
• past medical history
• time and mechanism of trauma
• initial eye, verbal, motor and pupillary responses
• other injuries
• clinical course

Brain death criteria

Performed by two independent doctors, one a consultant, the other a consultant or specialist registrar with 5 years post-registration experience.

Pre-conditions:

1 Confirm the underlying condition that resulted in irremediable brain damage.

2 Exclude the presence of cerebral depressants.

3 Exclude the presence of muscle relaxants.

4 Exclude metabolic or endocrine abnormalities.

5 Exclude hypothermia. Temperature should be $>35°C$.

Tests are positive (for brain death) if they confirm the absence of brain stem reflexes, i.e. there are:

no pupil responses
no corneal reflexes
no vestibulo-ocular reflexes
no motor responses within cranial nerve distribution to somatic stimulation of face, limbs or trunk
no gag or cough reflexes
no ventilatory efforts in the presence of a $PaCO_2 >6.7$ kPa (insufflate oxygen via suction catheter in tracheal tube).

Initial management of a patient with burns

A Airway. Give oxygen. Intubate trachea if airway in jeopardy or high level of suspicion of thermal injury to the airway.

B Breathing. IPPV for ventilatory failure, following inhalation injury, impaired consciousness, or signs of airway obstruction. Victims of carbon monoxide poisoning should receive 100% oxygen and hyperbaric therapy if available.

C Circulation. Insert two large bore i.v. cannulae away from burn site if possible. Take blood for U&E, FBC, and X-match. Site arterial cannula to take ABG and monitor arterial pressure directly.

Cutaneous burn results in the loss of temperature regulation. It is essential to resuscitate burned patients in a warm environment, using warmed fluids, warmed and humidified gases, and avoiding unnecessary exposure.

Control pain with bolus opioids and continue with an i.v. infusion.

Consider escharotomy or fasciotomy for tissue decompression and relief of ischaemia.

Give tetanus toxoid.

Estimation of burn size

Rapid assessment: 'Rule of nines' for adults (the body surface is divided into areas equivalent to ~9% each and the burned areas added together).

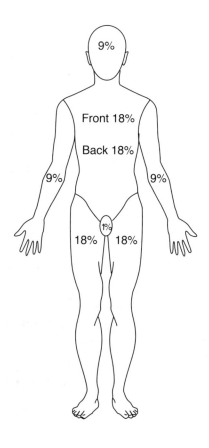

Note: The patient's palm surface area = approx. 1% BSA.
For a more accurate assessment of the surface area involved use the Lund and Browder chart (p. 79).

Fluid replacement regimens in burns

Fluid replacement regimens vary between centres and in different countries. Whichever regimen is used, the emphasis must be on regular assessment of the circulatory status and urine output (at least 1 ml kg^{-1} h^{-1}) and appropriate adjustment of the rate of fluid replacement made.

① REPLACEMENT BASED ON CRYSTALLOID

The volume of Ringer's solution in mls required in 24 h is:

4 ml kg^{-1} body weight (kg) × % surface area of burn

Half of this fluid volume is administered in the first 8 hours following the burn and the other half over the next 16 hours.

② REPLACEMENT BASED ON COLLOID

The volume of colloid in ml per time period required from the time of the burn is:

0.5–0.65 ml kg^{-1} × % surface area of burn

This volume should be given during **each** of the following time periods:

Time in hours from time of burn
0–4, 4–8, 8–12, 12–18, 18–24, 24–36

Note: *The volume of intravenous fluid required will be greater if the burns are not covered.*

Fluid replacement regimens in burns

Other formulae used to guide resuscitation include:

① PLASMA DEFICIT

The plasma deficit is derived from:

$$\text{Blood volume} - \left(\frac{\text{blood volume} \times \text{normal Hct}}{\text{observed Hct}} \right)$$

Note: *The normal blood volume of an adult is 75 ml kg^{-1}.*
The normal Hct of an adult female is 0.4, and 0.44 for a male.

② BLOOD REQUIREMENT

Blood is transfused in an adult when the calculated required volume exceeds 15% of the blood volume and in a child when it exceeds 10% of the blood volume. The volume to be replaced is calculated from:

1% normal blood vol. × % of full thickness burn

③ METABOLIC WATER REQUIREMENT

This is infused as 5% glucose over and above colloid requirement.

$$1.5\text{–}2 \text{ ml kg}^{-1} \text{ h}^{-1}$$

④ SODIUM REQUIREMENT

Expect to give 0.5 mmol kg^{-1} % burn^{-1} daily for the first few days.

Fluid replacement regimens in burns

6 CONSTITUENTS OF I.V. FLUIDS

Fluid	Na mmol^{-1}	K mmol^{-1}	Ca mmol^{-1}	Cl mmol^{-1}	HCO$_3$ mmol^{-1}	Glucose g l^{-1}
0.9% saline	150			150		
Hartmann's solution	131	5	2	111	29 (lactate)	
5% glucose						50
4% glucose with 0.18% saline	30			30		40
Haemaccel	145	5	6.2	145		
HAES-steril	154			154		
Gelofusine	154	0.4	0.4	125		
Hespan	154			154		
Dextran 70 in 0.9% saline	150			150		
Detran 70 in 5% glucose						50

Anaphylaxis

If the cause is obvious (e.g. a drug) discontinue the exposure. Then:

A   Airway
100% oxygen.

B   Breathing
Bag and mask ventilation, intubate if serious airway obstruction or if in cardiac arrest.

C   Circulation
i.m. adrenaline/epinephrine requires an effective circulation.

Age (years)	Volume of 1:1000 adrenaline/epinephrine (ml) given i.m.
<1	0.05
1	0.1
2	0.2
3–4	0.3
5	0.4
6–12	0.5
Adult	0.5 – 1.0

Intravenous adrenaline/epinephrine is preferred. The initial dose is:

$$50\text{–}100\ \mu g\ (0.5\text{–}1.0\ \text{ml of } 1{:}10\ 000)$$

Continue 100 μg boluses until hypotension and bronchospasm are corrected.

Anaphylaxis

An i.v. infusion of adrenaline/epinephrine or noradrenaline/norepinephrine may be needed:

> commence adrenaline/epinephrine or noradrenaline/norepinephrine at 0.025 µg kg^{-1} min^{-1} (see p. 17)
> give rapid i.v. fluid 10–20 ml kg^{-1}, preferably colloid.

Further management may include:

> salbutamol, 250 µg i.v. bolus then 5–20 µg min^{-1} infusion
> aminophylline, 5 mg kg^{-1} i.v. bolus over 20 min
> hydrocortisone, 500 mg i.v.
> chlorpheniramine, 20 mg i.v. diluted to 10 ml, given over 1 min
> sodium bicarbonate if severe acidosis persists.

Acute severe asthma

Features of life-threatening asthma include:

> silent chest
> cyanosis
> hypoxia
> inadequate ventilation
> unable to perform PEF
> bradycardia
> hypotension
> exhaustion
> confusion
> depressed level of consciousness
> acidosis
> raised or normal $PaCO_2$

Management comprises:

A Airway
Give oxygen.

B Breathing
Administer a β_2 agonist via oxygen driven nebuliser (e.g. salbutamol 5 mg or terbutaline 10 mg) continuously.

Hydrocortisone i.v. 200 mg 6 hourly (child:100 mg 6 hourly).

Aminophylline (may be given by bolus if the patient is not already taking theophylline) 5 mg kg^{-1} over 20 min. Consider a β_2 agonist i.v., e.g. salbutamol bolus 250 μg slowly followed by a salbutamol infusion at 3–20 μg min^{-1}, but more may be needed.

Acute severe asthma

B Breathing cont.

aminophylline maintenance infusion = 0.5 mg kg^{-1} h^{-1}
(child 6 months–9 years – 1.0 mg kg^{-1} h^{-1}
　　　　10–16 years – 0.8 mg kg^{-1} h^{-1}).

Ipratropium by nebulizer
　adult 0.5 mg
　child 0.25 mg (0.125 mg if very small).

Intubate and ventilate if deteriorating, or in the presence of impending exhaustion, despite maximal treatment.

C Circulation

Rehydrate with potassium-containing i.v. fluids.
NB: hypokalaemia may be severe.

CXR to exclude pneumothorax or pulmonary collapse.

Hypothermia

Management is determined by the degree of hypothermia.

Mild hypothermia (34–36°C):
Passive external rewarming.
Warm blankets, warm room.

Moderate hypothermia (30–34°C):
Passive rewarming.
Active rewarming of truncal areas.
Active internal rewarming.
Warmed i.v. fluids (to 43°C).
Warm humidified oxygen (42–46°C).

Severe hypothermia (<30°C)
Active internal rewarming.
Warm i.v. 0.9% saline (to 43°C).
Warm fluid lavage (43°C) potential sites:
peritoneum via dialysis catheter
bladder via urinary catheter
pleura via chest tube
oesophagus with oesophageal rewarming tubes
pericardium if open cardiac compression.
Warm humidified oxygen (42–46°C).
Ventilatory support.
Direct circulatory rewarming by arterio-venous bypass or cardiopulmonary bypass.

Note: *Defibrillation and cardiac drugs are unlikely to be effective at temperatures <30°C.*

Drug overdose

Your local poison centre: Tel. _____

Poison Information Services (UK and Ireland):

Belfast	01232 240503
Birmingham	0121 554 3801
Cardiff	01222 709901
Dublin	01 379964/6
Edinburgh	0131 229 2477
Leeds	0113 430715
London	0171 635 9191 or 0171 955 5095
Newcastle	0191 232 5131

GENERAL PRINCIPLES

A   Airway

Intubation is required if the laryngeal reflexes are obtunded.

B   Breathing

Oxygen.
IPPV for inadequate ventilation.

Consider the use of specific antagonists:
  Naloxone for narcotic overdose
  Flumazenil for benzodiazepine overdose.

C   Circulation

i.v. fluids to correct hypotension.
Vasopressor agents if hypovolaemia has been corrected but hypotension persists.
If arrhythmias occur ensure that hypoxia, hypercarbia, hypovolaemia, acidosis and electrolyte imbalances have been corrected.

Drug overdose

Consider the use of specific antagonists:
  Sympathomimetics in β-blocker overdose.
  Labetolol or esmolol for cocaine or amphetamine overdose.

Hypothermia (see p. 46)

Hyperthermia
Commence surface cooling and infuse cool i.v. fluids. Neuromuscular blockade, intubation and ventilation may be required. Dantrolene ($1\,mg\,kg^{-1}$ to a maximum of $10\,mg\,kg^{-1}$) may be of use in drug-induced hyperthermia, e.g. following amphetamine overdose.

Convulsions
Correct hypoxia, hypercarbia, hypovolaemia, acidosis, metabolic (including hypoglycaemia), and electrolyte imbalance. Treat with diazepam, 5–10 mg i.v. titrated to effect.

PREVENTING ABSORPTION

Gastric tubes and/or induced emesis should be avoided after ingestion of corrosives.

1 Emesis
Ipecacuanha:
  6–18 months old: 10 ml, older children: 15 ml,
  30 ml for adults, followed by 200 ml of water.

Contraindications to emesis:
  Inadequate laryngeal reflexes without the protection of tracheal intubation.
  Ingestion of petroleum derivatives and corrosives.

Drug overdose

2 **Gastric lavage**

3 **Activated charcoal**
Prevents absorption and promotes active elimination. The initial dose is 50 g orally, then 25 g every 4 h.

PROMOTION OF ELIMINATION

1 **Forced diuresis – alkaline**
This may be indicated for poisoning with:
barbiturates
salicylates
phenoxyacetate herbicides
and is achieved by administering the following fluids over 3 h.

> 500 ml 1.26% sodium bicarbonate
> 1000 ml 5% glucose
> 500 ml 0.9% saline + potassium chloride 20 mmol

2 **Forced diuresis – acid**
This may be indicated for poisoning with:
phencyclidine
amphetamine
fenfluramine
and is achieved by administering the following fluids at a rate of $1\,l\,h^{-1}$ for 4 h:

> 500 ml 5% glucose + 1.5 g ammonium chloride
> 500 ml 5% glucose
> 500 ml 0.9% saline

Drug overdose

3 **Peritoneal or haemodialysis**
This may be indicated for poisoning with:
    salicylates
    barbiturates
    methanol and ethanol
    ethylene glycol
    lithium.

4 **Haemoperfusion**
This may be indicated for poisoning with:
    salicylates
    barbiturates
    meprobamate
    disopyramide
    theophylline.

SPECIFIC ANTIDOTES

BENZODIAZEPINES
Flumazenil
100 µg increments titrated to effect.
Usual dose range 300–600 µg (max 2 mg).
Infusion 100–400 µg h^{-1}.

BETA-BLOCKERS
Glucagon
50–150 µg kg^{-1} i.v. bolus over 1 min, followed by an
infusion of 1–5 mg h^{-1}.

Isoprenaline
10–100 µg min^{-1} i.v. infusion titrated to effect.

Drug overdose

CYANIDE AND DERIVATIVES

Dicobalt edetate

600 mg by slow i.v. bolus over 1 min, followed by a further 300 mg if no response within 1 min.

Sodium nitrite

10 ml of 3% sodium nitrite i.v. over 3 min, followed by 25 ml of 50% sodium thiosulphate i.v. over 10 min.

DIGOXIN

Digoxin-specific Fab antibody fragments

IRON

Desferrioxamine

2 g in 10 ml sterile water i.m.

Gastric lavage with 2 g in 1000 ml warm water.

Leave 5 g in 50 ml water in stomach.

5 mg kg^{-1} h^{-1} given slowly by i.v. infusion (max 80 mg kg^{-1} day^{-1}),

or 2 g i.m. every 12 h.

METHANOL AND ETHYLENE GLYCOL

Ethanol

50 g orally or i.v., then 10–12 g h^{-1} to maintain a level of 1–2 g l^{-1} (higher rates are required for alcoholics and patients on dialysis).

OPIOIDS

Naloxone

0.4–2.4 mg i.v. repeated every few minutes to a total of 10 mg.

Drug overdose

PARACETAMOL

Acetylcysteine
150 mg kg^{-1} in 200 ml 5% glucose i.v. over 15 min;
then 50 mg kg^{-1} in 500 ml 5% glucose i.v. over 4 h;
then 100 mg kg^{-1} in 1000 ml 5% glucose i.v. over 16 h.
Total dose 300 mg kg^{-1} over 20 h.
Most effective when given within 8 h of ingestion.

Methionine
2.5 g 4 hourly for four doses (10 g over 24 h).

Paediatric resuscitation – ABC

The following pages contain key data for the resuscitation of the newborn, infant and child.

As with adults, when resuscitating neonates, or infants and children, adequate oxygenation and ventilation through a clear airway, chest compressions, and defibrillation are always more important than the administration of drugs.

Remember:

Call for help

ABC:
    Airway
    Breathing
    Circulation

Basic life support – newborn

1 Call for help from a person experienced in advanced resuscitation.

2 Position the baby flat or slightly head down.

3 Administer 100% oxygen via a funnel or ventilate with a face mask if apnoeic.

4 Commence external cardiac compressions if the heart rate is less than 60 min^{-1} or if pulse poor or absent. Compressions are performed using both thumbs. The neonate's chest is held between both hands and the thumbs placed over the junction of the middle and lower thirds of the sternum. The sternum is depressed smoothly and rhythmically by 2–3 cm.
The target rate of compressions is 120 min^{-1}.

5 Prevent heat loss. Dry the baby. Use warmed bedding and resuscitation surfaces. Keep the baby out of draughts. Resuscitate the baby under a radiant heat source. Maintain the ambient temperature at 24–25°C.

6 Neonates have a high glucose need and low glycogen store. During periods of stress the baby may become hypoglycaemic. Documented hypoglycaemia should be treated with an infusion of glucose.

Observe for:
a) symmetrical chest movement
b) onset of regular breathing
c) improvement in heart rate, peripheral perfusion, colour, movement, and tone.

7 Consider administering naloxone.

Acute perinatal blood loss

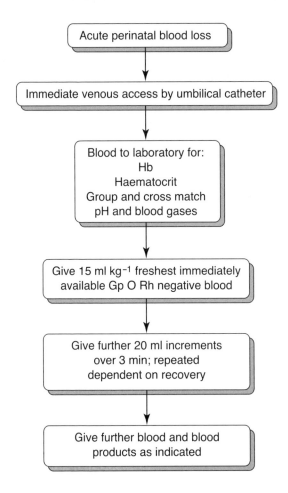

Acute perinatal blood loss

↓

Immediate venous access by umbilical catheter

↓

Blood to laboratory for:
Hb
Haematocrit
Group and cross match
pH and blood gases

↓

Give 15 ml kg⁻¹ freshest immediately
available Gp O Rh negative blood

↓

Give further 20 ml increments
over 3 min; repeated
dependent on recovery

↓

Give further blood and blood
products as indicated

Unanticipated meconium at delivery

1 Suck out the mouth and nose as soon as the head is delivered.

2 Call for help from a person experienced in advanced resuscitation.

3 Place the baby flat or slightly head down.

4 Suck out mouth and nose again.

5 Give oxygen by funnel.

6 If meconium aspiration is suspected proceed to direct laryngoscopy (see p. 57).

Meconium aspiration

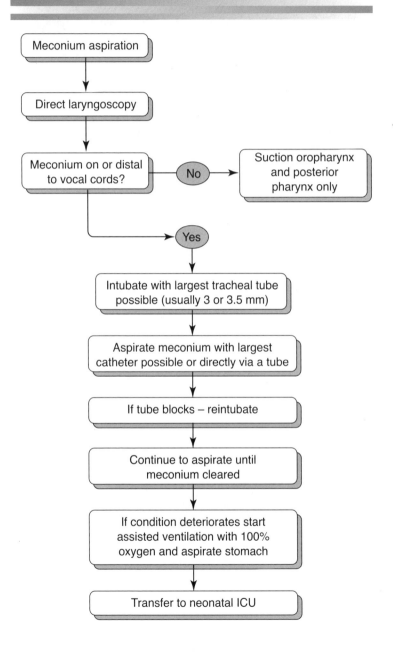

Meconium aspiration

↓

Direct laryngoscopy

↓

Meconium on or distal to vocal cords? — No → Suction oropharynx and posterior pharynx only

Yes

↓

Intubate with largest tracheal tube possible (usually 3 or 3.5 mm)

↓

Aspirate meconium with largest catheter possible or directly via a tube

↓

If tube blocks – reintubate

↓

Continue to aspirate until meconium cleared

↓

If condition deteriorates start assisted ventilation with 100% oxygen and aspirate stomach

↓

Transfer to neonatal ICU

P
A
E
D
I
A
T
R
I
C

Apgar score

	0	1	2
Heart rate	Absent	Slow (<100)	>100
Respiratory effort	Absent	Weak cry, hypoventilating	Crying lustily
Muscle tone	Flaccid	Some flexion of limbs	Well flexed
Colour	Blue or white	Blue hands or feet	Healthy pink
Reflex irritability	No response	Some movement	Active movement

Note: *The Apgar score is assessed at 1 and 5 minutes after birth. The maximum score is 10.*

Basic life support – infants and children

The following guidelines apply to infants and children under the age of 8 years. Large or older children should be resuscitated as described for adult victims (p. 31).

VENTILATION

The target tidal volume for a child is sufficient to see the chest rise and fall.

The target rate for a victim who is not breathing but who has a pulse is 20 breaths per minute.

Inflation should take about 1.5 seconds.

If the victim is not breathing and has no pulse, two effective breaths should be given before starting chest compressions and then one breath after every five compressions.

If you have difficulty achieving an effective breath:
➠ Recheck the child's mouth and remove any obstruction
➠ Ensure adequate head tilt/chin lift (but do not over extend)
➠ Make up to five attempts to achieve at least 2 effective breaths
➠ If still unsuccessful, move on to choking sequence (p. 62).

Basic life support – infants and children

CHEST COMPRESSIONS

These are performed over the lower half of the sternum.

The target rate of compressions is at least 100 per minute.

The sternum should be depressed by about a third of the depth of the child's chest.

Pressure should be applied vertically and smoothly with the compressed and relaxed phases being of equal duration.

Continue resuscitation until:

⟴ The child shows signs of life
⟴ Qualified help arrives
⟴ You become exhausted.

Paediatric basic life support

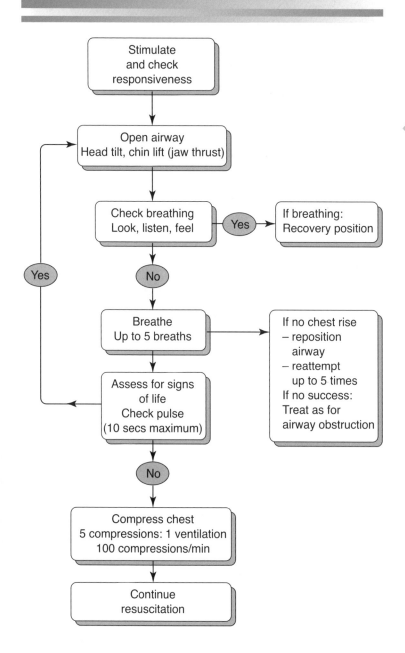

Choking – infant

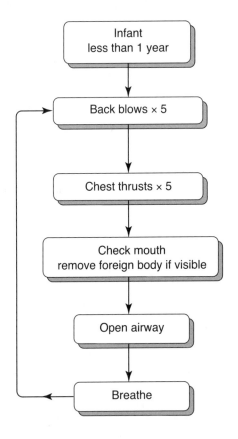

Notes: **Back blows.** The infant or child is held prone and five smart blows delivered to the middle of the back between the shoulder blades. The head must be below the level of the chest during this manoeuvre.

Chest thrusts. The child is placed in a supine position with the head lower than the chest. Chest thrusts are administered in a similar way to chest compressions except that thrusts are sharper and more vigorous and are carried out at a rate of 20 per minute.

Abdominal thrusts are not performed in this age group as there is the risk of visceral rupture.

Choking – child

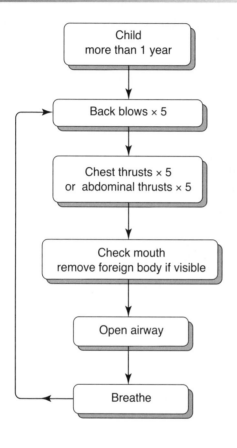

Child
more than 1 year

↓

Back blows × 5

↓

Chest thrusts × 5
or abdominal thrusts × 5

↓

Check mouth
remove foreign body if visible

↓

Open airway

↓

Breathe

Notes: ***Abdominal thrusts.*** *Administer five abdominal thrusts after 10 back blows (2 × 5) have been delivered. Use the upright position (Heimlich manoeuvre) if the child is conscious. An unconscious child should be laid supine and the heel of one hand placed in the middle of the upper abdomen. Five sharp thrusts should be directed upwards towards the diaphragm.*

The choking treatment algorithm should be continued until the foreign body is cleared or the child breathes spontaneously.

Paediatric advanced life support

The following pages contain treatment recommendations presented as algorithms.

These algorithms are not intended to replace clinical understanding or prohibit flexibility.

Cardiac arrest in children has a much worse outcome than in adults. In adults cardiac arrest is primarily cardiac in origin. In children cardiac arrest is usually secondary to failure of other organs. Respiratory failure is the most common cause of cardiac arrest in children, the second most common being circulatory failure due to loss of circulating volume. Early recognition of respiratory and circulatory failure are thus the key to improving survival. Establishing a clear airway, providing oxygenation, ensuring an adequate circulating volume, and directing specific treatment to the underlying cause are the priorities of resuscitation.

Asystole is the most common arrest rhythm in children and is usually preceded by bradycardia. Ventricular fibrillation is uncommon in children, it is therefore inappropriate to include a precordial thump or series of DC shocks unless VF is confirmed on ECG.

Paediatric advanced life support

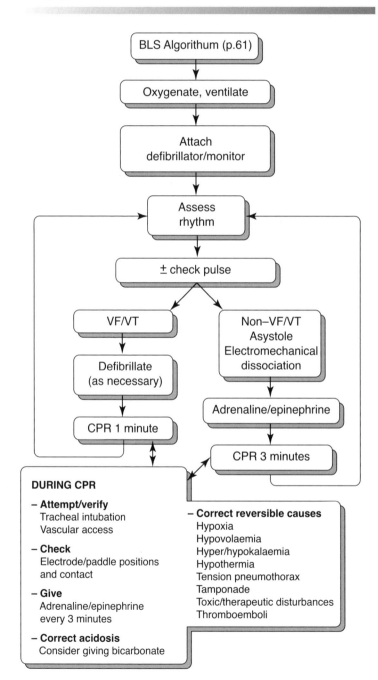

BLS Algorithm (p.61)

↓

Oxygenate, ventilate

↓

Attach defibrillator/monitor

↓

Assess rhythm

↓

± check pulse

VF/VT

↓

Defibrillate (as necessary)

↓

CPR 1 minute

Non–VF/VT
Asystole
Electromechanical dissociation

↓

Adrenaline/epinephrine

↓

CPR 3 minutes

DURING CPR

– **Attempt/verify**
Tracheal intubation
Vascular access

– **Check**
Electrode/paddle positions
and contact

– **Give**
Adrenaline/epinephrine
every 3 minutes

– **Correct acidosis**
Consider giving bicarbonate

– **Correct reversible causes**
Hypoxia
Hypovolaemia
Hyper/hypokalaemia
Hypothermia
Tension pneumothorax
Tamponade
Toxic/therapeutic disturbances
Thromboemboli

Non-VF/VT

This is more common in children than VF/VT.

If venous or intraosseous access secured, give
   10 μg kg^{-1} adrenaline/epinephrine
   (0.1 ml kg^{-1} of 1:10 000 solution)

If no venous or intraosseous access, consider
   100 μg kg^{-1} adrenaline/epinephrine via tracheal tube
   (1 ml kg^{-1} of 1:10 000 solution)

Perform 3 minutes of CPR.

If venous or intraosseous access secured, give
   100 μg kg^{-1} adrenaline/epinephrine
   (1 ml kg^{-1} of 1:10 000 solution)

VF/VT

This is unusual in children.

Defibrillation

The initial three shocks are delivered at
  $2\,J\,kg^{-1}$, $2\,J\,kg^{-1}$, $4\,J\,kg^{-1}$.

All shocks thereafter are delivered at $4\,J\,kg^{-1}$.

Paediatric resuscitation chart

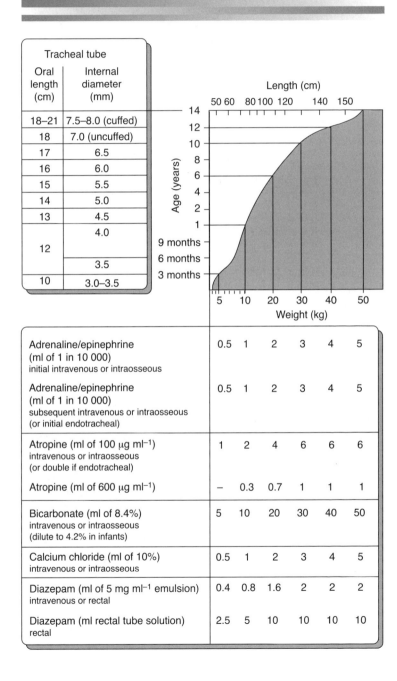

Tracheal tube	
Oral length (cm)	Internal diameter (mm)
18–21	7.5–8.0 (cuffed)
18	7.0 (uncuffed)
17	6.5
16	6.0
15	5.5
14	5.0
13	4.5
12	4.0
	3.5
10	3.0–3.5

Length (cm)

50 60 80 100 120 140 150

Age (years)

14 12 10 8 6 4 2 1

9 months
6 months
3 months

5 10 20 30 40 50

Weight (kg)

Adrenaline/epinephrine (ml of 1 in 10 000) initial intravenous or intraosseous	0.5	1	2	3	4	5
Adrenaline/epinephrine (ml of 1 in 10 000) subsequent intravenous or intraosseous (or initial endotracheal)	0.5	1	2	3	4	5
Atropine (ml of 100 μg ml⁻¹) intravenous or intraosseous (or double if endotracheal)	1	2	4	6	6	6
Atropine (ml of 600 μg ml⁻¹)	–	0.3	0.7	1	1	1
Bicarbonate (ml of 8.4%) intravenous or intraosseous (dilute to 4.2% in infants)	5	10	20	30	40	50
Calcium chloride (ml of 10%) intravenous or intraosseous	0.5	1	2	3	4	5
Diazepam (ml of 5 mg ml⁻¹ emulsion) intravenous or rectal	0.4	0.8	1.6	2	2	2
Diazepam (ml rectal tube solution) rectal	2.5	5	10	10	10	10

Paediatric resuscitation chart

Tracheal tube	
Oral length (cm)	Internal diameter (mm)
18–21	7.5–8.0 (cuffed)
18	7.0 (uncuffed)
17	6.5
16	6.0
15	5.5
14	5.0
13	4.5
12	4.0
	3.5
10	3.0–3.5

Glucose (ml of 50%) intravenous or intraosseous (dilute to 25% in infants)	5	10	20	30	40	50
Lignocaine (ml of 1%) intravenous or intraosseous	0.5	1	2	3	4	5
Naloxone neonatal (ml of 20 μg ml^{-1}) intravenous or intraosseous	2.5	5	–	–	–	–
Naloxone adult (ml of 400 μg ml^{-1})	–	0.25	0.5	0.75	1	1.25
Salbutamol (mg nebuliser solution) by nebuliser (dilute to 2.5–5 ml in physiological saline)	–	2.5	5	5	5	5
Initial DC defibrillation (J) by ventricular fibrillation or pulseless ventricular tachycardia	10	20	40	60	80	100
Initial DC cardioversion (J) for supraventricular tachycardia with shock (synchronous or ventricular tachycardia with shock (non-synchronous)	5	5	10	15	20	25
Initial fluid bolus in shock (ml) crystalloid or colloid	100	200	400	600	800	1000

Paediatric resuscitation chart

Note: *Non-standard drug concentrations may be available for some of the agents.*

Atropine: Use 100 µg ml^{-1} by diluting 1 mg to 10 ml or 600 µg to 6 ml in 0.9% saline.

Calcium: 1 ml of calcium chloride 10% is equivalent to 3 ml calcium gluconate.

Lignocaine: Use 1% or give twice the volume of 0.5% or half the volume of 2%, or dilute appropriately.

Salbutamol: may also be given by slow i.v. infusion but beware the different concentrations available (e.g. 50 and 500 µg ml^{-1}).

Paediatric trauma – principles

The same priorities of assessment and management that apply to adults also apply to victims of paediatric trauma (p. 25).

Key points to remember in paediatric trauma are:

1 Children often show cardiorespiratory compensation until precipitous collapse.

2 High surface area to body mass ratio results in an increased potential for heat loss. It is thus essential to resuscitate children in a warm environment, using warmed fluids, warmed and humidified gases, and avoiding unnecessary exposure.

3 The high compliance of the paediatric skeleton results in internal organ injury in the absence of obvious overlying surface injury.

4 If an emergency surgical airway becomes necessary, needle cricothyroidotomy and jet insufflation is preferred to surgical cricothyroidotomy because of the risk of laryngeal injury with the latter.

5 CT scanning offers an alternative to diagnostic peritoneal lavage for assessing abdominal trauma provided it is immediately available and does not interrupt the resuscitative process.

6 Failure to cannulate a vein after two attempts in shocked children aged less than 6 years is an indication to proceed to intraosseous infusion.

Paediatric vital signs

An estimate of a child's normal systolic blood pressure can be made using the formula:

$$\text{blood pressure (mmHg)} = 80 + (\text{age} \times 2)$$

Children have a greater circulatory physiological reserve than adults. By comparison with adults, signs of impending circulatory collapse may be only slight despite considerable blood loss. The diagnosis of shock, or its precursors, in children is made on the appearance of the skin, the capillary refill and temperature of the extremities, and the presence of an altered cerebral state. Fluid resuscitation should not be withheld until the vital signs are abnormal.

	Age		
	<1 year	2–5 years	5–12 years
Heart rate (beats min^{-1})	120–140	100–120	80–100
Blood pressure (systolic) (mmHg)	70–90	80–90	90–110
Respiratory rate (breaths min^{-1})	30–40	20–30	15–20
Blood volume (ml kg^{-1})	90	80	80

Paediatric resuscitation formulae

The following formulae provide rapid estimates.

Body weight (kg)

  1–8 years: (Age × 2) + 9
  8–13 years: Age × 3

Tracheal tube internal diameter (mm)

$$(Age/4) + 4.5$$

This is approximately the same size as the child's nostril or little finger.

Tracheal tube length (cm)

  Oral: (Age/2) + 12
  Nasal: (Age/2) + 15

Maintenance fluid requirement (per kg body weight)

0–10 kg: $4 \text{ ml kg}^{-1} \text{ h}^{-1}$

11–20 kg: $4 \text{ ml kg}^{-1} \text{ h}^{-1}$ for the first 10 kg
     + $2 \text{ ml kg}^{-1} \text{ h}^{-1}$ for the remainder

>20 kg: $4 \text{ ml kg}^{-1} \text{ h}^{-1}$ for the first 10 kg
     + $2 \text{ ml kg}^{-1} \text{ h}^{-1}$ for the second 10 kg
     + $1 \text{ ml kg}^{-1} \text{ h}^{-1}$ for the remainder

Intraosseous infusion

This is a suitable means of administering fluid to children aged less than 6 years in whom venous cannulation has failed.

A 16 or 18G bone marrow needle is inserted into the tibia on its anteromedial surface 1–3 cm below the tibial tubercle. The needle is directed inferiorly to avoid the epiphyseal plate. In the presence of tibial fractures the distal femur may be used.

The following have been successfully administered by the intraosseous route:

Crystalloid fluids
Colloid fluids
Blood
Adrenaline/epinephrine
Antibiotics
Atracurium
Atropine
Calcium
Dobutamine
Dopamine
Digoxin
Glucose
Lignocaine
Midazolam
Sodium bicarbonate
Suxamethonium

It should be expected that virtually all drugs may be given by this route.

Paediatric fluid administration

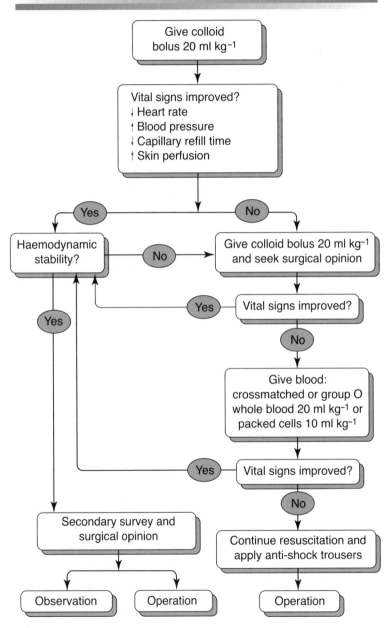

Give colloid
bolus 20 ml kg⁻¹

Vital signs improved?
↓ Heart rate
↑ Blood pressure
↓ Capillary refill time
↑ Skin perfusion

Yes   No

Haemodynamic
stability?   No   Give colloid bolus 20 ml kg⁻¹
and seek surgical opinion

Yes   Vital signs improved?

Yes   No

Give blood:
crossmatched or group O
whole blood 20 ml kg⁻¹ or
packed cells 10 ml kg⁻¹

Yes   Vital signs improved?

No

Secondary survey and
surgical opinion

Continue resuscitation and
apply anti-shock trousers

Observation   Operation   Operation

Note: *The use of paediatric anti-shock trousers is controversial in
some centres.*

75

Paediatric trauma score

	+2	+1	−1
Weight	>20 kg	10–20 kg	<10 kg
Airway	Normal	Oral or nasal airway	Intubated
Blood pressure	>90 mmHg	50–90 mmHg	<50 mmHg
Level of consciousness	Completely awake	Obtunded or any LOC*	Comatose
Open wound	None	Minor	Major or penetrating
Fractures	None	Minor	Open or multiple

*LOC = loss of consciousness.

Notes: The paediatric trauma score (PTS) assesses child size, airway, systolic blood pressure, level of consciousness, cutaneous and skeletal injury.

Children with a PTS <8 should be managed in institutions with the facilities and experience to deal with major paediatric trauma.

Children with scores >8 have the highest potential for preventable morbidity and mortality and require close observation and monitoring.

Paediatric Glasgow coma score

		>1 year	<1 year	
Eye opening	4	Spontaneously	Spontaneously	
	3	To verbal command	To shout	
	2	To pain	To pain	
	1	No response	No response	
Best motor response	5	Obeys commands		
	4	Localizes pain	Localizes pain	
	3	Flexion to pain	Flexion to pain	
	2	Extension to pain	Extension to pain	
	1	No response	No response	

		>5 years	2 – 5 years	0 – 2 years
Best verbal response	5	Orientated and converses	Appropriate words and phrases	Smiles and cries appropriately
	4	Disorientated and converses	Inappropriate words	Cries
	3	Inappropriate words	Cries	Inappropriate crying
	2	Incomprehensible sounds	Grunting	Grunting
	1	No response	No response	No response

Normal aggregate score:

<6 months	12	2–5 years	14
6–12 months	12	>5 years	14
1–2 years	13		

Initial management of a paediatric patient with burns

The same general principles apply to the management of a child with burns as those used in the treatment of burned adults (p. 37). However, a more accurate assessment of the percentage body surface area involved is required in children and the method described by Lund and Browder may be used (p. 79).

The adequacy of fluid replacement is monitored by ensuring a urine output of at least 1 ml kg^{-1} h^{-1} in children aged over 1 year and at least 2 ml kg^{-1} h^{-1} in those under 1 year.

Because of the small diameter of the paediatric airway, any evidence of airway injury should result in a rapid respiratory assessment and a low threshold for early tracheal intubation.

Cutaneous burn results in the loss of temperature regulation. This, combined with the high surface area to body mass ratio of a child results in an increased potential for heat loss. It is thus essential to resuscitate burned children in a warm environment, using warmed fluids, warmed and humidified gases, and avoiding unnecessary exposure.

Paediatric burns – assessment of surface area

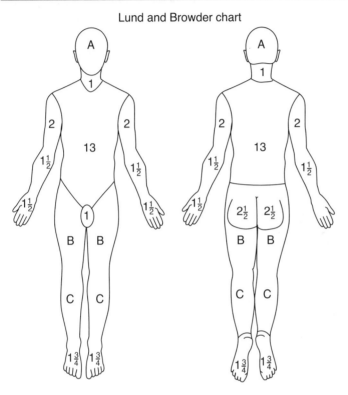

Lund and Browder chart

Relative percentage of body surface area affected by growth

Area	Age (years)					
	0	1	5	10	15	Adult
A = $\frac{1}{2}$ of head	$9\frac{1}{2}$	$8\frac{1}{2}$	$6\frac{1}{2}$	$5\frac{1}{2}$	$4\frac{1}{2}$	$3\frac{1}{2}$
B = $\frac{1}{2}$ of one thigh	$2\frac{3}{4}$	$3\frac{1}{4}$	4	$4\frac{1}{2}$	$4\frac{1}{2}$	$4\frac{3}{4}$
C = $\frac{1}{2}$ of one leg	$2\frac{1}{2}$	$2\frac{1}{2}$	$2\frac{3}{4}$	3	$3\frac{1}{4}$	$3\frac{1}{2}$

Haematology

	Neonate	**Child**	**Adult**
Hb (g dl^{-1})	18–19	11–14	13.5–17.5 (M) 11.5–15.5 (F)
Hct	0.55–0.65	0.36–0.42	0.4–0.45 (M) 0.36–0.44 (F)
MCV (fl)	100–125	80–96	83–96
MCHC (g l^{-1})	30–34	32–36	32–36
WBC ($\times$ 10^9 l^{-1})	6–15	5–14	4–11
Neutrophils (% of WBC)	30–50	40–70	50–75

Note: Equivalent umbilical cord blood values are:
Hb 13.5–20 g dl^{-1}, Hct 0.5–0.56, MCV 110–128 fl, MCHC 29.5–33.5 g l^{-1}, WBC 9–30 $\times$ 10^9 l^{-1}, neutrophils 50–80%.

Coagulation

Platelet count ($\times 10^9$ l^{-1})   150–400

Bleeding time (min)   <7

Prothrombin time (sec)   11.5–15

Activated partial thrombo-plastin time (sec)   25–37

Thrombin time (sec)   10

Fibrinogen (g l^{-1})   2–4.5

FDPs (mg l^{-1})   <10

Biochemistry

	Neonate	Child	Adult
Na (mmol l^{-1})	130–145	132–145	133–143
K (mmol l^{-1})	4.0–7.0	3.5–5.5	3.6–4.6
Cl (mmol l^{-1})	95–110	95–110	95–105
Cr (μmol l^{-1})	28–60	30–80	60–100
Urea (mmol l^{-1})	1.0–5.0	2.5–6.5	3–7
Mg (mmol l^{-1})	0.6–1.0	0.6–1.0	0.7–1
Ca (mmol l^{-1})	1.8–2.8	2.15–2.7	2.25–2.7
Phosphate (mmol l^{-1})	1.3–3.0	1.0–1.8	0.85–1.4
Bilirubin (μmol l^{-1})	<200	<15	<17
Alkaline phosphatase (U l^{-1})	150–600	250–1000	21–120
AST (U l^{-1})	<100	<50	6–35
Total protein (g l^{-1})	45–75	60–80	62–80
Albumin (g l^{-1})	24–48	30–50	35–55
Globulin (g l^{-1})	20–30	20–30	22–36

Blood gases

ARTERIAL

pH	7.34–7.46
PaO$_2$ (kPa [mmHg])	10–13.3 [75–100]
PaCO$_2$ (kPa [mmHg])	4.4–6.1 [33–46]
Actual bicarbonate (mmol l^{-1})	22–26
Standard bicarbonate (mmol l^{-1})	22–26
Base excess	± 2
Oxygen saturation	0.96–1.0

MIXED VENOUS

pH	7.32–7.42
PaO$_2$ (kPa [mmHg])	4.96–5.6 [36–42]
PaCO$_2$ (kPa [mmHg])	5.3–6.9 [40–52]
Oxygen saturation	0.7–0.8

Conversion factors

1 mmHg = 133.3 Pa = 1.36 cmH$_2$O = 1.25 cm blood

100 mmHg = 13.3 kPa

760 mmHg = 101.3 kPa

1 kPa = 7.5 mmHg = 10.2 cmH$_2$O

1 mmH$_2$O = 0.073 mmHg

100 kPa = 15 psi

1 atm = 1 Bar = 101.3 kPa = 1033 cmH$_2$O

Bibliography

Advanced Life Support Working Party of the European Resuscitation Council, 1994. Peri-arrest arrhythmias (management of arrhythmias associated with cardiac arrest). *Resuscitation,* 1994; **28**:151–159.

Advanced Life Support Working Party of the European Resuscitation Council, 1994. Peri-arrest arrhythmias: notice of 1st update. *Resuscitation,* 1996; **31**:281.

Baskett P J F. *Resuscitation Handbook* (2nd ed.). London: Mosby Year Book, 1993.

Baskett P J F, Strunin L, eds. Resuscitation. *British Journal of Anaesthesia,* 1997; **79** (2).

Conference of the Medical Royal Colleges and their Faculties. Diagnosis of brain death. *British Medical Journal,* 1976; **2**:1187–1188.

European Resuscitation Council. *Resuscitation,* 1998; **37** (2). In press.

Grande C M, ed. *Textbook of Trauma Anesthesia and Critical Care.* St Louis: Mosby Year Book, 1993.

Lloyd-Thomas A R. Paediatric trauma: primary survey and resuscitation – II. *British Medical Journal,* 1990; **301**:380–382.

Lund C C, Browder N C. The estimation of areas of burns. *Surgery, Gynecology & Obstetrics,* 1944; **79**:352–358.

Bibliography

Recommendations of the 1992 National Conference. Guidelines for cardiopulmonary resuscitation and emergency cardiac care. *The Journal of the American Medical Association*, 1992; **268**:2171–2302.

Skinner D, Driscoll P, Earlam R, eds. *ABC of Major Trauma*. London: British Medical Association, 1991.

Index

Index

Index